Leaky Gut Solution: How to Cleanse and Detoxify your Body of Leaky Gut Syndrome Quickly and Effectively

Table of Contents

Introduction

Human body is made of number of numerous small and big organs that work together as a system. Each of these organs plays a specific role in the body and operates in co-ordination with other systems. When all of these parts function properly, a person is healthy and fit. There are several factors that determine how healthy a person is, but the most important factor is the food he eats. What goes into the stomach of a person directly influences how he feels and how it affects the body. So, it is not surprising when somebody says that health of the gut determines the overall health of the body.

With the progress of medical science, there is diagnosis and cures available for some of the most life threatening diseases. But, some discussions and conditions are still under debate in the medical community; one of them is whether Leaky Gut Syndrome exists or not. Though opinions over it a divided, and so are ways in which it can be treated, awareness about Leaky Gut Syndrome is growing slowly.

When someone mentions bacteria, people generally perceive them to be harmful to the body. But that's not the case. There are bacteria that are required by the body and functioning of the body will not be possible without them. The human gut alone consists of millions of good bacteria that help in processing food, assisting in digestion and producing anti-bodies to strengthen immune system. If the friendly bacteria get outnumbered by harmful bacteria, a person starts feeling sick, has digestive problems, fatigue and other issues. This condition may be due to Leaky Gut Syndrome. Difficult to diagnose with absence of unique symptoms, Leaky Gut Syndrome directly influences immune system of the body. Bad food, improper eating habits and stressful modern lifestyle are three main reasons behind this syndrome. Discovering and isolating Leaky Gut Syndrome is essential as it may evolve into serious, life threatening diseases if left untreated.

What is Leaky Gut Syndrome

One of the commonly discussed terms and rapidly growing conditions these days is Leaky Gut Syndrome. A medical condition, it is still considered to be a concept that is being researched on for its legitimacy. But, growing cases of people suffering from similar problems and recognizable conditions of the disease are bringing a change to the way doctors and other people in medical community perceive Leaky Gut Syndrome. This syndrome is related to the small intestine and the lining inside this body organ. In medical term, Leaky Gut Syndrome is described as 'Hyperpermeable Intestines'.

In the human body, each organ is designed to perform a specific function that contributes to the proper functioning of the body. Small intestine is a part of the digestive system of the body and is very important as it absorbs nutrients from food. Most of the minerals and vitamins from food a person eats regularly are absorbed in the small intestine. For absorption of these nutrient elements, the intestine has a lining of mucosal cells. These mucosal cells contain microscopic pores that act like filter and transfer nutrients into blood and discards toxic elements. Presence of pores makes walls of the intestine semi-permeable. In simple terms, semi-permeable means the lining of intestinal tract is like a net with minute holes in it. As these holes are extremely small, lining in gut acts as a barrier and keeps out bigger particles from entering into bloodstream. If these big size particles are allowed to enter bloodstream, they can cause damage to functioning of other systems in body. So, with digestive lining, certain elements from food pass and enter the bloodstream while other elements are blocked. Blood carries and deposits these nutrients in all parts of the body.

In case of Leaky Gut Syndrome, the gut lining of intestine get damaged and permeability also increases. This results in bigger holes in the net, thus compromising barrier for particles entering the system. With the damaged net and bigger holes, undigested food particles, viruses, bacteria and toxic waste products enter into the bloodstream. These are then transported to all parts of the body and trigger reaction from immune system.

Why is It a Mystery

The biggest reasons why Leaky Gut Syndrome is mysterious and not openly accepted by medical community is the lack of definite symptoms and conditions. It is still considered to be a psychological syndrome by many and is not portrayed as a medical ailment in medical schools too. It is still a confusing condition with very limited awareness about it, its treatments, ways of diagnosis and therapies that can be used to treat it.

Symptoms of Leaky Gut Syndrome are not exclusive and unique. Similar symptoms are visible in a number of other commonly found medical problems, hence it is difficult to pinpoint to any symptom and state that it is a symptom of Leaky gut Syndrome. Similarly, there are no exclusive tests that can uncover a definite problem as this syndrome. Without a proper diagnosis, this syndrome is left undiagnosed and untreated in most cases. Thus, even if a person's health has been significantly affected and weakened, it is difficult to say that it is due to Leaky Gut Syndrome.

How is It Caused

The term 'Leaky Gut Syndrome' itself is under debate, and so are its symptoms and solutions. How Leaky Gut Syndrome is caused and how it affects the system of body is not certain with people having very little clue about it. The only thing known is that it causes pores of intestinal lining to widen and leads to leakage of toxins in bloodstream.

But, leaky gut syndrome can get very serious; hence it is important to know factors that can cause this syndrome. Causes of Leaky Gut Syndrome includes –

- **Food with Toxic Chemicals** – Presence of preservatives and pesticides in food introduces lot of chemicals into the body. These chemicals are actually toxins that trigger reactions in the body. Not just preservatives, there are chemicals present in processed foods, flavorings, artificial sweeteners and refined sugar also.

- **High Intake of Grains and legumes** - Whole grains contain gluten which increase permeability of intestinal muscles. Similarly, legumes also contain some anti-nutrients that may cause damage and inflammation of intestinal tract.

- **Improper Chewing of Food** – If the food is not chewed properly, it affects the digestion process and breakdown of food into proteins. As more protein gets released into the system, it causes damage to normal digestive process.

- **Yeast** – When taken in a high quantity, yeast develops into a fungus that clings to the intestinal lining. If this multi-celled fungus is allowed to stay on the lining, it makes it permeable and results in big holes.

- **Deficiency of Zinc** – Out of all minerals required for body, zinc is mainly required for regulating strength of intestinal lining. So, deficiency of zinc weakens gut lining, reduces its integrity and makes it permeable.

- **Chronic Stress** – Modern lifestyle and chronic levels of stress have a great influence on the immune system. More the level of chronic stress, more suppressed the immune system becomes. If the immune system performs less than normal, it results in inflammation of gut lining and increased permeability of the tract.

- **Modern Lifestyle** – Modern day lifestyle has altered eating and living habits, and not all changes have positive influence on body. Increase consumption of processed products, late work nights, improper sleep and eating schedules, increase consumption of alcohol and other habits directly or indirectly influence the immune system.

- **High Dose of Anti-inflammatory Medicines** – High dose of anti-biotics and anti-inflammatory drugs can cause damage to the intestinal lining.

Symptoms of Leaky Gut Syndrome

Symptoms of any disease help in identifying it, and taking necessary actions to curb and heal it. But, in case of Leaky Gut Syndrome, the symptoms are still not clear and very diverse. There are no specific set of symptoms that point towards this problem. The only warning sign you must look out for is allergies. If a person is experiences different type of sensitivities to food, there is a high chance he is suffering from Leaky Gut Syndrome. Commonly found symptoms of this medical problem includes –

- Sensitivity to multiple food products

- Problems in digestive system

- Bowel diseases

- Inflammation in body frequently

- Pain in joints

- Conditions related to thyroid

- Nasal congestion or sinus

- Bloating

- Unexplainable gain in weight

- Issues related to skin and skin allergy like rash

- Headaches and migraines

- Hives

- Fungal disorders

- Mood swings and depression

- Mental fog and tiredness

Diseases that can develop due to Leaky Gut Syndrome

Leaky Gut Syndrome may not be a chronic ailment, but it is left diagnosed it can trigger evolution of several life threatening diseases and problems. Research have found that Leaky Gut Syndrome has resulted in onset of various diseases like –

- Arthritis

- Asthma

- Obesity

- Cancer

- Celiac and other autoimmune diseases

- Eczema or psoriasis

- Type 1 diabetes

- Heart failure

- Chronic fatigue

- Parkinson's disease

- Alzheimer's disease

- Multiple Sclerosis

- Ulcers

- Infections from parasites

- Autism

- Fibromyalgia

Solutions to Leaky Gut Syndrome

Causes of Leaky Gut syndrome are still a mystery, with constant research being conducted on causes and remedies for the same. But, this does not mean that people expect a miracle to treat their problem. Leaving Leaky Gut Syndrome unattended will not only worsen the condition but also trigger new and more serious ailments in the body.

There is no thumb-rule or a set of defined steps to treat Leaky Gut Syndrome. But there are small things, small changes in lifestyle and diet that help in restoring a healthy gut. Plan your diet in a way that reduces inflammation of intestinal tract and improves its integrity. Here are some solutions for treating Leaky Gut Syndrome -

- In Leaky Gut syndrome, diet plays an influential role. Hence, it very important to have a balanced diet regularly. The body requires more energy for rapid conversion of food hence, it is better to include energy boosting food in your regular diet.

- First step to heal Leaky Gut syndrome is to smoothen the digestive process and stabilize digestive process. To completely detox and cleanse the body, avoid allergens like soy, alcohol, yeast, sugar, legumes, grains and other food products initially till the gut is healthy.

- Cleansing of body includes cleansing of bowel, liver and kidney. Cleansing is required to remove toxins and parasites. You can opt for professional cleansing problems or make changes to your diet that trigger cleansing naturally.

- Remember, your digestive processes are influenced by your thoughts. Relax your mind before you start with your lunch/dinner.

- Leaky Gut Syndrome results in improper digestion of food, hence there is a high probability that the person suffers from specific nutritional deficiencies. So, first get a checkup for vital nutrients and take specific supplements in case of deficiency.

- Assess your daily diet and analyze foods that are damaging your gut. Replace these foods with foods that help in healing your gut.

- Inflammation triggering foods cause the most damage to intestinal tract, hence avoid such foods in all forms. It includes artificial sweeteners, refines sugar, alcohol, gluten-rich food and others.

- Water intake is as vital as proper food intake as water plays an important role in digestion of food. You should drink at least 2 liters of water every day.

- Don't have your food in a hurry or gulp it down. Chew your food properly; it must almost turn into a liquid before you swallow it down.

- Proper combination of food is as important as proper food intake. Avoid food pairing like oil and fruits, sweet and proteins and other similar combinations that affect digestion process. Practice implementing proper food combinations in diet.

- Include liquid in various forms in your diet along with plain water. You can have warm water with lemon, fruit juices, thin almond milk or any other form of water.

- Include fiber-rich foods, especially fermentable fibers, in your meals as they are important for balancing friendly bacteria in body. Fermentable fibers can be in the form of yam, sweet potato, yucca and others.

- Limit the amount of caffeine, recreational drugs and caffeine in your daily diet. Avoid them as much as possible.

- Avoid soda or other kinds of frizzy drinks as they can cause bloating of stomach.

- Opt for organic and pesticide-free fruits and vegetables as pesticides are one of the top toxic elements for a leaky gut.

- Increase the proportion of raw food in your diet in form of salads. Try to have as much raw vegetables and fruits as you can as it increases enzymes helpful in breaking down of food. Enzymes from raw food also act as garbage collectors in body by removing damaged mucosal cells, bacteria and toxins from body.

- Rebalance the quantity of probiotics in your diet. Introduce different forms of probiotic food in your regular meals. Probiotic food have bacteria stop inhabitance of bad bacteria in body, hence you need to make sure that there is a continuous supply of probiotics to body. Bacteria from probiotics also help in food absorption, healing of intestinal gut line and keep check on vicious cycle of bacteria growth.

- Adding Vitamin D to the diet in form of multi-vitamins helps in removing irritants and bringing intestinal lining to normal.

- Avoid vegetables like eggplants, tomatoes, potatoes, all types of peppers. Instead opt for colorful vegetables like cabbage, cauliflower, kale and green leafy vegetables.

- Try to consume fruits like berries that are high in anti-oxidants and minerals.

- Include 5-8 servings of fresh vegetables and fruits in your diet regularly along with high quality protein.

- Limit the consumption of nuts excluding macadamias and coconut.

- Avoid foods that irritate the gut, including egg whites.

- Omega 3 is known to have highly beneficial effects on intestinal lining, hence, try to include fish oil in your diet. If you are vegetarian or vegan, look for alternate sources of Omega 3.

- Avoid refined, deodorized or polyunsaturated oils instead use healthy oils like olive oil or coconut oil.

- Vitamin D is very important for a healthy gut. Hence, spend time in early morning sun everyday as well as look for food sources that are rich in Vitamin D.

- Balanced diet does not necessarily meal having full meals three times a day and that too every day. Keep altering your food habits and bring innovation to your diet chart. You can keep some days as liquid only days while follow some days as fat-free days.

- Include amino acid rich food in your every meal as amino acids help in reducing inflammation and regulating digestive system.

- Stay away from cigarettes completely.

- Watch out for food that trigger allergies or conditions like diarrhea or irritation in bowel. Every person may have an allergy to a different food, so analyze the pattern. If you always feel sick after consuming a particular vegetable or dairy product, you may be allergic to it. Try to exclude such foods from your diet as much as you can.

- Get tests done to verify presence of intestinal pathogens in the body. If these parasites are present, get them treated immediately.

- Try to include foods that heal intestinal tract naturally instead of taking synthetic or artificial therapies.

- If you have questions regarding food planning or diet sources, consult a nutritionist and seek their help.

- Modern lifestyle, especially stress, is a major reason for development of Leaky Gut Syndrome. So, find ways to lower and manage your stress levels.

- Indulging in physical activity or workout regularly also helps in cleansing the body and managing stress. You can choose any exercise form you are comfortable with whether it is a morning jog, aerobics or dancing.

- Remember, never exercise or workout with a full stomach.

- Sweating is another effective way for cleansing the body and washing away toxins in body. Try to include workout, running, cycling or other sweat producing exercise forms regularly in your schedule. You can also cleanse your body by sweating with sauna or drinking warm tea in a hot temperature room.

- Get good quality and sufficient sleep daily as it is important for managing stress level.

Foods Beneficial for Digestive Health

For a healthy gut, you need to have a healthy digestive system. What a person eats, his habits and lifestyle is directly related to his digestive well being, which in turn influences the Leaky Guts Syndrome. Just like a person needs to avoid certain foods when diagnosed with Leaky Gut Syndrome, there are several food products that he should consume. Foods that benefits healing of intestinal track and digestive health –

- **Kefir** – Probiotic in nature, Kefir is basically a drinkable form of yoghurt. As it is fermented, it provides the body with friendly bacteria that helps production of enzymes and heals the immune system. Make sure that the Kefir you are consuming has limited content of sugar as too much of sugar will destroy the bacteria.

- **Products made from Coconut** – Whether you consume coconut oil or coconut milk, it is really beneficial for your intestine and immune system. Fat content of coconut oil is very less while other coconut products help in reducing bacteria, fungus and other irritants in intestine.

- **Bone Broth** – Soup or broth made from bones of duck, fish, chicken, turkey or any other animal are very beneficial for healing damaged gut lining. This broth contains nutrients as well as anti-inflammatory properties that help in strengthening intestinal tract.

A healthy gut is the key to a healthy life! So, no doubt, you need to make sure that you keep your gut healthy and ailment free. A minor infection in the gut if left ignored can cause bigger problems later on. Not just physical health, gut is responsible for your mental well being too. In this fast-paced life, people tend to overlook their health needs and issues till they don't become very serious. With the number of people falling prey to chronic diseases increasing, it has become very important for people to pay attention to their health. Staying healthy is not tough; you simply need to alter some habits in your lifestyle. Not only does what you drink and eat affect your digestive health, but what you think has an influence on your health too. Eat healthy, think healthy and stay healthy!